YOUR KNOWLEDGE HAS VALUE

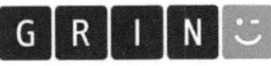

Bibliographic information published by the German National Library:

The German National Library lists this publication in the National Bibliography; detailed bibliographic data are available on the Internet at http://dnb.dnb.de .

Imprint:

Copyright © 2018 GRIN Verlag
Print and binding: Books on Demand GmbH, Norderstedt Germany
ISBN: 9783668677258

This book at GRIN:

https://www.grin.com/document/418814

Vinod Nair Sreekumar

Osseointegration. A Critical Appraisal

GRIN Verlag

GRIN - Your knowledge has value

Since its foundation in 1998, GRIN has specialized in publishing academic texts by students, college teachers and other academics as e-book and printed book. The website www.grin.com is an ideal platform for presenting term papers, final papers, scientific essays, dissertations and specialist books.

Visit us on the internet:

http://www.grin.com/

http://www.facebook.com/grincom

http://www.twitter.com/grin_com

Table of Contents

1

1. Introduction

Osseointegration of dental implants Dental implantology, a special field of dentistry dealing with the rehabilitation of the damaged chewing apparatus due to loss of the natural teeth, is currently the most intensively developing field of dentistry. Missing teeth can be replaced by dental implants (artificial roots), which are inserted into the root-bearing parts of the mandible or maxilla. The success and long-term prognosis of implant prosthetic therapy depend primarily on the anchorage of the implant in the jawbone, i.e. on the osseointegration. Today, there are ever increasing demands from patients with missing teeth for masticatory function and aesthetic appearance of their replaced teeth to be restored and for shortening of the period of osseointegration of the implants, which takes a relatively long time (3-6 months). The successful insertion of a biocompatible material into living tissue with little to no evidence of rejection has revolutionized medicine and dentistry.

In the 1960s, Brånemark et al. stumbled upon this phenomenon when using titanium (Ti) in animal models, with little idea of the impact this discovery would have on the rehabilitation of future medical and dental patients. This phenomenon, described as "osseointegration", was characterized by a number of clinical and ultra-structural observations. Osseointegration may broadly be defined as the dynamic interaction and direct contact of living bone with a biocompatible implant in the absence of an interposing soft tissue layer [1-3].

Although the clinical term osseointegration describes the anchorage of endosseous implants to withstand functional loading, it provides no insight into the mechanisms of bony healing around such implants. However, in the last decade it became clear that the long-term success of dental implants also depends on the complex bio integration of these alloplastic materials, which is determined by the responses of the different surrounding host tissues (the alveolar bone, the conjunctival part of the oral soft tissues and the gingival epithelium). Critical in developing biologic design criteria for implant surfaces is to understand the sequence of bone-healing events around endosseous implants is believed to be Bone growth on the implant surface can be subdivided into three distinct phases that can be addressed experimentally [4].

The first, osteoconduction, relies on the migration of differentiating osteogenic cells to the implant surface, through a temporary connective tissue scaffold. The second, de novo bone formation, results in a mineralized interfacial matrix, equivalent to that seen in cement lines in natural bone tissue, being laid down on the implant surface. The implant surface topography determines whether the interfacial bone formed is bonded to the implant. A third tissue response, the bone remodelling, creates a bone-implant interface comprising de novo bone formation. Treatment outcomes in dental implantology depend critically on the implant surface designs that optimize the biological response during each of these three distinct integration mechanisms.

Today, much effort is devoted to the design, synthesis and fabrication of Ti dental implants in order to obtain long term (lifelong) secure anchoring in the bone. Fundamentally, this means the ability of then implant to carry and sustain the dynamic and static loads that it is subjected to. The bulk structure of the material governs this ability. Evidently, it is important to achieve a proper function in the shortest possible healing time, with a very small failure rate and with minimal discomfort for the patient. These factors are also important for cost reasons. As regards osseointegration, i.e. the formation of a direct connection between the living bone and the surface of the load-carrying implants, the important question arises as to how to attain a better integration by modification of the implant surface morphology.

A wide variety of materials have been used to produce endosseous implants [5, 6]. Currently, Ti and its alloys are the most commonly utilized dental and orthopaedic implant materials that meet the most important requirements [7, 8]. The properties of Ti and its surface, which is covered by a native oxide layer, are appropriate to allow its use as a biocompatible material [9]. At a cellular level, the relationship of an implant with the surrounding tissue is highly dependent on the interaction between the passive titanium oxide (TiO2) which is formed on the surface of a Ti implant, and biological elements such as collagen, osteoblasts, fibroblasts and blood constituents [2,10]. The TiO2 layer is very stable, corrosion-resistant and may be manipulated to have variable thickness. The clinician is often faced with the challenge of identifying the successful osseointegration of a dental implant. Clinical success is determined by a lack of mobility and by the ability of the implant to resist functional loading (chewing force) without mechanical deformation and to transfer the load onto the alveolar bone without deterioration of the bony interface [11].

Radio graphically, the bone should appear to be closely apposed to the implant surface. The resolution currently achievable in medical imaging, however, is several orders of magnitude less than what is required to observe a soft tissue cell. Accordingly, radiographic assessment alone is unsuitable to determine with certainty whether a soft tissue is present [12]. A number of studies have analysed this bone to Ti interface histologically and ultrastructurally, often with inconsistent findings. The difficulty arises primarily with the need to prepare and section the specimens without changing or damaging the interface. Recent studies have utilized CT scanning to obtain a 3-dimensional picture of the implant interface [13, 14].

2. Biomaterials used in guided bone regeneration (GBR)

The aesthetic and functional demands of the patients have recently increased enormously. In dental implantology, new biomaterials and available surgical techniques furnish excellent possibilities. However, there are certain fundamental weaknesses in the current technology. Patients must have suitable morphology and a sufficient amount of available jawbone for reconstruction to be a viable option. After extraction or the loss of teeth for any other reason, the edentulous alveolar ridge resorbs. Consequently, its dimensions and morphology, especially as concerns the labial plate, rapidly become inadequate for the appropriate accommodation of artificial roots. To preserve the height and width of the alveolar bone for future implantation therapy, guided tissue regeneration (GTR) procedures are used [15].

GBR has become a routinely applied method in dental implantology. Most of the dentoalveolar regenerative techniques require osteoconductive material in order to establish new bone formation in the necessary anatomical form. This surgical procedure makes use of barrier membranes to direct the growth of new bone at sites having insufficient volumes or dimensions for function or prosthesis placement. GBR is similar to any other GTR utilized in dental therapy, but is focused on the development of bony tissues instead of soft tissues of the periodontal attachment. Used in conjunction with a sound surgical technique, GBR is a reliable and validated procedure [16]. Xenograft bone substitutes originate from a species other than human, e.g. bovine. Xenografts are usually distributed only as a calcified matrix. Bio-Oss is a safe, effective xenograft: a deproteinized, sterilized bovine bone with 75-80% porosity. It is reported to be highly osteoconductive and biocompatible. It is known that Bio-Oss serves as a scaffold in GBR, but, due to its poor resorbability, it may exert a negative influence on the structure of the newly formed bone. The large-mesh interconnecting pore system facilitates angiogenesis and the migration of osteoblasts. It has been found clinically that its resorption is very similar to that of human bone [17-19]. Pure beta-tricalcium phosphates (TCP-β) such as Cerasorb are widely used osteoconductive materials. The chemical characteristics of Cerasorb allow it to resorb completely and quite rapidly during new bone formation. This may result in too early resorption in some cases without fulfillment of the clinical requirement of the space-maintaining function [20, 21].

These bone-substitute materials allow targeted bone regeneration as they facilitate construction of a base on which implants can be positioned and further stabilized. Cerasorb has good osteoconductive and resorption properties [21, 23]. Full resorption over a defined period of time, with simultaneous transformation into autologous bone, is of particular significance in this respect. Because of its rounded surface and chemical composition, Cerasorb is remarkably bio inert and is therefore particularly suitable for innovative procedures. The unique open porosity structure increases active cellular in-growth and improves nutrition, while the rough surface further increases osteoconductivity. The result is the rapid in-growth of local bone and a significantly shorter resorption time (6-12 months) compared with other ceramic products [22].

Calcium phosphate cements (CPCs, e.g. Vitalos) are an emerging class of bone-substitute materials that are capable of rapid setting to a hard mass, providing a scaffold for the bone remodelling process. The CPCs synthetic bone graft materials invented in the 1980s, consist basically of tricalcium phosphate and anhydrous dicalcium phosphate. Many different combinations of calcium and phosphate have been developed as commercial CPC materials [24]. Hydroxyl-apatite (HA) is the main component of VitalOs and the primary inorganic component of natural bone which makes the hardened cement biocompatible and osteoconductive. Over time, CPC is gradually resorbed and replaced by new bone. CPC has two significant advantages over pre-formed, sintered ceramics.

First, CPC paste can be sculpted during surgery to fit the contours of the wound. Second, the nanocrystalline HA structure of the CPC makes it osteoconductive, causing it to be gradually resorbed and replaced by new bone. Recent work with CPCs has focused on improving the mechanical properties, making premixed CPCs, giving the CPCs macro porous properties and seeding cells and growth factors into the cement [25]. CPCs are identified as alloplastic materials appropriate for osseous augmentation because of the unique combination of Osseo conductivity, biocompatibility, mouldability and malleability.

In contrast with conventional bone graft materials, CPCs can be directly moulded and shaped to fill intrabony defects. Moreover newly-developed CPCs are fully injectable, which ensures easy handling and appropriate application of these materials [26].

3. Surface modifications of Ti implants to improve osseointegration

The biological responses of the surrounding tissues to dental implants are controlled largely by their surface characteristics (chemistry and morphology). The biorecognition takes place at the interface of the implant and host tissue [27]. Biological tissues interact mainly with the outermost atomic layers of an implant, which measure about 0.1-1 nm. The molecular and cellular events at the bone-implant interface are not yet fully understood and there are still some uncertainties concerning the molecular structure of the bone-implant interface [28, 29]. The rationale for the surface modification of implants is straightforward: to retain the key physical properties of an implant, while modifying only the outermost surface layer to influence the bio-interaction. As a result, much research work is devoted to the elaboration of methods of modifying surfaces of existing implants (biomaterials) in order to achieve the desired biological responses. These responses can be several: in a healthy patient it may be a regular osseointegration process, but an older or even an ill patient a smaller bone quantity or a not ideal bone quality means a handicap in bio integration. These cases are often avoided by appropriate patient selection. As the length of the average human lifetime is increasing, more and more people are living with missing teeth and in widely differing status of health. There is a demand at present for the optimization of Osseo/bio integration processes (reducing the 3-6-month healing period) even for people in different status of health. For dental implants, as for other biomaterials, the bio- and osseointegration processes can be controlled at molecular and cellular levels by modification of the implant surface. There are various surface-modification possibilities, which are usually subdivided into physicochemical and biochemical methods [28].

4. Physicochemical methods

The most common physicochemical treatments are chemical surface reactions, e.g. oxidation, acid-etching, sand-blasting, ion implantation, laser ablation, surface coating with calcium phosphate, etc. These methods alter the energy, charge and composition of the existing surface, but can lead to surfaces with modified roughness and morphology. The surface energy plays an important role not only with regard to protein adsorption, but also as concerns cell attachment and spreading [30]. The surface charge influences both the molecular or cellular orientation and the cellular metabolic activity [31]. The roughness of the implant surface plays a significant role in anchoring cells and connecting together the surrounding tissues, thereby leading to a shorter healing period. These surfaces display advantages over smooth ones as the area of contact is enlarged by micro structuring the implant surface.

Acid-etching, sand-blasting and Ti plasma-spraying are typical methods for the development of rough surfaces and are well documented with in vitro and in vivo methods [32-35]. Ion implantation methods are generally used to improve the mechanical quality of an implant. For example iridium has been ion implanted in the Ti-6Al-4V alloy to improve its corrosion resistance [36] and the implantation of nitrogen into Ti reduces wear significantly [37]. To increase the roughness of solid surfaces, a number of laser-based techniques have been applied in the last decade [38]. The advantages of using lasers for the ablation of surfaces are the precise control of the frequency of the light, the wide range of frequencies available, the high energy density, the ability to focus and raster the light, and the ability to pulse the source and control the reaction time. Lasers commonly used for surface modification include ruby, Nd: YAG, argon, CO2 and excimer [39, 40].

Besides the prompt intense heating of the surface, excimer laser illumination may further enhance the sterilizing effect in consequence of the high dose in the UV range [41]. Inorganic materials, such as the bio reactive calcium phosphate (CaP) coatings (or HA), have been extensively applied because of their chemical similarity to bone minerals. Several studies have shown that these coatings achieve a very intimate contact between the implant and bone [42, 43]. Clinical investigations have reported a high degree of success with HA-coated implants, with a reduction of the healing period [44].

However, in other studies, HA-coated implants showed signs of the covering material peeling off from the implant surface, which may induce foreign body reactions [45, 46]. Furthermore, a long-term clinical study of HA-coated oral implants indicated a significantly lower survival rate (77.8% after 8 years) for HA-coated implants as compared with TPS-coated (Ti-plasma-sprayed) implants (92.7%) [47]. The biodegradation of these coatings may be the reason why HA coatings are no longer the surface modifications of choice.

5. Biochemical methods

For implants, the goal of biochemical methods is to immobilize peptides, proteins and enzymes on the surface in order to induce specific cell and tissue responses (adhesion, signalling and stimulation) and to control the tissue-implant interface with molecules delivered there directly [28]. Numerous different biologically functional molecules can be immobilized onto Ti surfaces to enhance bone regeneration at the interface of implant devices. One essential aspect is the maintenance of the bioactivity (or the recognizable binding site) of these molecules during their incorporation into a biomimetic coating. CaP coatings and the purely organic components of bone can serve as carrier systems for osteogenic drugs, thereby rendering them osteoinductive and osteoconductive.

The most promising candidates for osteogenic agents are the members of the transforming growth factor-β (TGF-β) superfamily, such as bone morphogenic proteins (BMPs). Following its successful coprecipitation with the inorganic components and incorporation, BMP-2 retains its biological activity in vitro [48]. The application of BMPs to improve the present implantation techniques appears rather promising [49, 50]. BMPs such as rhBMP-2 (recombinant human BMP-2) are growth factors that could be employed to augment the resorbed alveolar ridge prior to implantation. BMP-2 is a member of the TGF-β superfamily of multifunctional cytokines. Mature BMP2 is a homodimer of two subunits, each consisting of 114 peptides [49]. The two chains are held together by a single disulphide group. The monomers contain six additional cysteine residues, which are involved in three intrachain disulphide linkages. The cysteine residue is characteristic of all members of the TGF-β superfamily [51].

The molecular structure of rhBMP-2 BMPs induce bone formation and regeneration, and thereby play important roles in repair processes. BMP-2 exhibits high osteoinductive properties as it attracts osteoprogenitor cells and directs their differentiation into osteoblasts. When used in conjunction with implants, BMPs form a monolayer on the surface of the device, which causes cell proliferation, thereby increasing the incorporation of the device. Overall, the main effect of BMPs (including rhBMP-2) is the stimulation of bone growth through an increase in cell differentiation [52, 53]. At present, four major strategies exist for organic coating approaches: immobilization of extracellular matrix (ECM) proteins (collagen, etc.) or peptide sequences as modulators for bone cell adhesion, deposition of cell signalling agents (bone growth factors) to trigger new bone formation, immobilization of DNA for structural reinforcement and enzyme-modified Ti surfaces for enhanced bone mineralization [48].

Biomolecules can be immobilized by physical absorption (van der Waals or electrostatic interactions), physical entrapment (use of barrier systems) and covalent attachment. The selection of the immobilization method depends on the working mechanism of the specific biomolecules, which dictates, for instance, a short-term, transient immobilization for growth factors and a longterm immobilization for adhesion molecules and enzymes. The cell membrane receptor family of integrin's is involved in cell adhesion to ECM proteins. These integrins bind to specific amino acid sequences within ECM molecules and in particular to the RGD (arginine-glycine-asparagine) sequence. For this reason, the most commonly used peptide sequence for surface modification is the above-mentioned cell adhesion motive [54, 55]. PE film coatings modify the solid/liquid interface in such a way as to ensure a suitable environment for the adsorption of proteins. The alternating adsorption technique has been successfully applied in different fields of science, as a consequence of its numerous practical applications. It can be automated, it involves the use of aqueous solutions, it is environment-friendly, and various substrates can be covered with films of readily variable thickness [56].

In consequence of its structural properties, DNA is of high potential for application as a biomaterial coating, regardless of its genetic information. Additionally, DNA can be used as a drug delivery system since its functional groups allow the incorporation of growth factors. The studies by van den Beucken et al. [57] proved that DNA-based coatings improve the deposition of CaP. A relatively new approach for surface modification is enzyme-modification of the Ti surface to enhance bone mineralization along the implant surface. In particular the enzyme alkaline phosphatase (AP) is known to increase the local concentration of inorganic phosphate, and to decrease the concentration of extracellular pyrophosphate, a potent inhibitor of mineralization [58]. In the past decade, another viable biomimetic strategy has appeared: organic-inorganic composite coatings. These mimic the bone structure, which is composed of an organic matrix (90% of which comprises collagenous proteins) and an inorganic CaP phase. Collagen-CaP [59], growth-factor-CaP [60] and PE multilayers-CaP [61] composite coatings have been developed and have furnished promising in vitro and in vivo experimental results.

Many of the above-mentioned biochemical methods are still in the experimental stage and the in vivo applications (animal or clinical studies) are still ahead. It is believed that these surfaces will make an enormous positive contribution to clinical implant science, especially if the older subjects or patients are targeted.

6. Animal models for the investigation of osteogenesis and osseointegration

Researchers often use laboratory animals as models of humans. The use of animal models in oral health science has increased significantly over the past 20 years. In attempts to understand the onset and dissemination of different oral diseases and to identify and develop dental materials and methods suitable for the restoration of the damaged tissues, animal experiments are of fundamental significance. A specific model is chosen because it is believed to be appropriate to the condition being investigated and is thought likely to respond in the same way as humans to the proposed treatment for the character being investigated. After the model has been chosen, it is essential that any experiments in which it is used are well designed, i.e. are capable of demonstrating a response to any treatment applied. If the model happens to be insensitive or the experiments are badly designed (e.g. the use of too few animals) so that they are incapable of distinguishing between the treated and control groups, the model is not appropriate for its purpose. When new animal experiments are introduced five key features of the animal models used in biomedical research must be considered [62-64]

1. There can be substantial asymmetry between the model and the target in the numbers of similarities and differences. In theory, the model and the target only need to have a single feature in common, but there can be any number of differences. This means that useful models can sometimes be highly abstract, such as a mathematical equation or computer simulation. Moreover, the more fundamental the biological process, the more likely it is that the animal model and humans will respond similarly.

2. Some differences between the model and the target are necessary; otherwise the animal would not be a model. Differences are as important as similarities as they allow us to do things with the model which would not be possible with a human. Mice are widely used because they are 12 small and prolific, and their genetics can be manipulated in ways not possible with humans. These differences from humans make them more, not less, valuable as models of

10

humans for some applications. Characteristics such as a small size may make them unsuitable for other applications, e.g. heart surgery or bone surgery.

3. Models are highly specific to a particular study. Strains of mice and rats which develop cancer, heart disease, diabetes or neurological diseases could be of great interest in the study of these diseases, but these animals would probably be unsuitable for regulatory toxicology, where long-lived strains are usually required. Thus, it is impossible to say whether the rat for example, is a good or bad model of humans without specifying the context of the proposed study.

4. Models need to be validated. Research using animal models usually aims at the prediction of a response in humans. When a new treatment for a particular disease or condition is developed in animals, clinical trials will normally show whether or not the model was valid. If not, it may either be because the model was biologically invalid, or because the experiments in which the model was utilized were badly designed.

5. Models are subject to improvement through further research. Much of animal research is aimed at achieving an understanding of the animal as a potential model for particular human conditions. Models are not simply found: they need to be developed, and this requires an understanding of the biology of the species and the effects of various interventions. In investigations of the osseointegration of dental implants and different biomaterials, successful research is seldom limited to an anatomical region, such as the soft and hard tissues of the mouth. Relevant models are often used to answer more general biological questions.

To study bone formation and or osseointegration with the application of the maxillofacial region, the long bones and the calvarias are often used, and not only the jawbones. Bone is a highly differentiated tissue. After an injury, there is a possibility that bone will heal not as bone, but as fibrous connective tissue. Undue heat injury increases this risk of disturbed bone healing. During surgical interventions in bone, frictional energy generates heat, and thereby increases the risk of fibrous bone healing. This basic knowledge is of utmost significance in all animal experiments involving bone cutting and drilling. The most often used and preferred animal models for investigations of the osseointegration of dental implants and the osteogenesis of different bone substitutes are the rabbit femur and tibia models [65, 66].

Although this model is easy to handle and has made a significant contribution to our studies, it presents disadvantages, too. The main drawback of this model is that, as the femur is a long bone, the new bone is formed according to endochondral ossification (a cartilage model serves as the precursor of the bone), unlike in the skull. The flat bones of the skull and face, the mandible and the clavicle are developed by intramembranous ossification. This is a simpler method, without the intervention of a cartilage precursor. It is emphasized that these concepts (intramembranous and endochondral ossification) refer only to the mechanism by which a bone is initially formed. Because of the rapid bone remodelling that occurs during bone development, the initial bone tissue laid down by intramembranous or endochondral formation is quickly replaced. The replacement bone is established on the pre-existing bone by appositional growth and is identical in both cases. Another disadvantage of this rabbit femur or tibia model is that, due to the relatively thin cortical bone width, during the operative drilling or after the postoperative healing period there is a risk of unwanted pathological fractures, especially if the drilling is bicortical (e.g. an implant inserted through the width of the long bone), not monocortical.

In view of these disadvantages of the rabbit femur model, my goal was to develop a new animal model in rabbit and pig calvarial bones. Calvarial wound models bear many similarities to the maxillofacial region. Both calvarial and midfacial bones develop from a membrane precursor, and the calvaria and mandible consist of two cortical tables with regions of intervening cancellous bone. It contains modest amounts of bone marrow, which generally facilitates bone formation, although bone marrow is not indispensable for bone formation. When the aim is to investigate the pattern of bone formation in growth areas, young animals in an intense craniofacial growth period are preferably used.

In adult animals, the regenerative capacity of the cranium is reduced; this therefore constitutes a suitable site for research work on agents for the enhancement of bone repair. Small defects (5 mm in diameter) that would correspond to a typical operative defect in clinical maxillofacial surgery have been produced and used in rats and rabbits. This size makes spontaneous bone regeneration possible, allows an evaluation of the regenerative influence stemming from the implant material and of the maturation of the newly formed bone, and permits tests on several implant materials. A critical-size defect is a defect that will not heal during the lifetime of the animal. When a defect large enough to preclude spontaneous healing is employed, the osteogenic potential of an implant or a graft may be considered unambiguous. The critical-size model allows an assessment of whether enhancement of bony regeneration occurs [67-72].

7. Conclusion

In modern implantology, the need for bone augmentation techniques demands adequate osteoinductive and osteoconductive effects from the bone substitutes. It is very important that the original form of the bone should be reconstructed and also that an appropriate bone structure should be achieved as soon as possible. Bio-Oss is a highly osteoconductive xenograft material certified for the regeneration of bone defects. In our experiments, we found that it displays very low resorbability and acts as an inert scaffold onto which bone-forming cells and blood vessels creep, forming the new bone. In conclusion, Cerasorb seemed to have good bioresorptive and osteoconductive properties.

References

[1] Branemark P, Zarb G, Albrektsson T: Tissue-Integrated Prostheses Osseointegration in Clinical Dentistry. Chicago, Quintessence Publishing Co. Inc. 1985

[2] Albrektsson T, Hansson H, Kasemo B, Larsson K, Lundstrom I, McQueen D, Skalak R: The interface of inorganic implants in vivo; titanium implants in bone. Annals of Biomedical Engineering 1983, 11:1-27.

[3] Masuda T, Yliheikkila P, Felton D, Cooper L: Generalizations Regarding the Process and Phenomenon of Osseointegration. Part I. In Vivo Studies. The International Journal of Oral and Maxillofacial Implants 1998, 13:17-29.

[4] Davies J: Mechanisms of Endosseous Integration. International Journal of Prosthodontics 1998, 11:391-401.

[5] Williams DF: Implants in dental and maxillofacial surgery. Biomaterials 1981; 2:133-136.

[6] Lemons JE: Dental implant biomaterials. J Am Dental Assoc 1990; 121:716-719.

[7] Brånemark PI, Adell R, Albrektsson T, Lekholm U, Lundkvist S, Rockler B: Osseointegrated titanium fixtures in the treatment of edentulousness. Biomaterials 1983, 4:25–28

[8] Meffert RM, Langer B, Fritz ME: Dental implants: a review. J Periodontol 1992, 63:859–870

[9] Lautenschlager EP, Monaghan P: Titanium and titanium alloys as dental materials. Int Dental J 1993, 43:245–253.

[10] Schroeder A, Van der Zupen E, Stich H, Sutter F: The Reactions of Bone, Connective Tissue and Epithelium to Endosteal Implants with Titanium Sprayed Surfaces. Journal of Oral and Maxillofacial Surgery 1981, 9:15-25.

[11] Zarb G, Albrektsson T: Guest Editorial: Osseointegration: A Requiem for the Periodontal Ligament? The International Journal of Periodontics & Restorative Dentistry 1991, 11:88-91.

[12] Albrektsson T, Johansson C, Sennerby L: Biological aspects of implant dentistry: osseointegration. Periodontology 2000, 4:58-73.

[13] Akagawa Y, Wadamoto M, Sato Y, Tsuru H: The three-dimensional bone interface of an osseointegrated implant: A method for study. The Journal of Prosthetic Dentistry 1992, 68:813-816.

[14] Wadamoto M, Akagawa Y, Sato Y, Kubo T: The three-dimensional bone interface of an osseointegrated implant. I: A morphometirc evaluation in initial healing. The Journal of Prosthetic Dentistry 1996, 76:170-175.

[15] Lynch SE, Genco RJ, Marx RE: Tissue Engineering: Applications in Maxillofacial Surgery and Periodontics, Quintessence Publishing Co, Inc. 1999

[16] Buser D, Bornstein MM, Weber HP, Grütter L, Schmid B, Belser UC: Early implant placement with simultaneous guided bone regeneration following single-tooth extraction in the esthetic zone: a crosssectional, retrospective study in 45 subjects with a 2- to 4-year follow-up. J Periodontol 2008, 79:1773-81.

[17] Hämmerle CHF, Chiantella GC, Karring T, Lang NP: The effect of a deproteinized bovine bone mineral on bone regeneration around dental implants. Clin Oral Implant Res 1998, 9:151-162.

[18] Orsini G, Traini T, Scarano A, Degidi M, Perrotti V, Piccirilli M, Piattelli A: Maxillary sinus augmentation with Bio-Oss particles: A light, scanning, and Transmission Electron Microscopy study in man, J Biomed Mater Res Part B: Appl Biomater 2005, 74B:448-457.

[19] Jensen SS, Broggini, N, Hjørting-Hansen E, Schenk R, Buser D: Bone healing and graft resorption of autograft, anorganic bovine bone and β-tricalcium phosphate. A histologic and histomorphometric study in the mandibles of minipigs. Clin Oral Implant Res 2006, 17:237-243.

[20] Suba Z, Takács D, Gyulai–Gaál S, Kovács K: Facilitation of β-tricalcium phosphate-induced alveolar bone regeneration by platelet-rich plasma in beagle dogs: a histologic and histomorphometric study. Int. J. Oral Maxillofac. Implants 2004, 19:832-838.

[21] Suba Zs, Takács D, Matusovits D, Barabás J, Fazekas A, Szabó Gy: Maxillary sinus floor grafting with β-tricalcium phosphate in humans: density and microarchitecture of the newly formed bone. Clin. Oral Impl. Res. 2006, 17:102-108.

[22] Zerbo IR, Bronckers ALJJ, de Lange G, Burger EH: Localization of osteogenic and osteoclastic cells in porous β-tricalcium phosphate particles used for human maxillary sinus floor elevation. Biomaterials 2005, 26:1445-1451.

[23] Hoshino M, Egi T, Terai H, Namikawa T, Takaoka K: Repair of long intercalated rib defects using porous beta-tricalcium phosphate cylinders containing recombinant human bone morphogenetic protein-2 in dogs. Biomaterials 2006, 27:4934-4940.

[24] Friedman CD, Costantino PD, Takagi S, Chow LC: BoneSource hydroxyapatite cement: a novel biomaterial for craniofacial skeletal tissue engineering and reconstruction. J Biomed Mater Res 1998; 43:428–32.

[25] Brown GD, Mealey BL, Nummikoski PV, Bifano SL, Waldrop TC: Hydroxyapatite cement implant for regeneration of periodontal osseous defects in humans. J Periodontol 1998; 69:146–57.

[26] Xu HH, Quinn JB, Takagi S, Chow LC: Processing and properties of strong and nonrigid calcium phosphate cement. J Dent Res 2002; 81:219–24.

[27] Kasemo B: Biological surface science. Surface Science 2002, 500:656–677.

[28] Puleo DA, Nanci A: Understanding and controlling the bone-implant interface. Biomaterials 1999, 20:2311-2321.

[29] Klinger MM, Rahemtulla F, Prince CW, Lucas LC, Lemons JE: Proteoglycans at the bone-implant interface. Crit Rev Oral Biol Med 1998, 9:449-463.

[30] Baier RE, Meyer AE: Implant surface preparation. Int J Oral Maxillofac Implants 1988, 3:9-20.

[31] Meyle J: Cell adhesion and spreading on different implant surfaces. In Lang N, Karrig T, Lindhe J. Proceedings of the 3rd European Workshop on Periodontology, Quintessenz Verlags-GmbH, Berlin, 1999

[32] Buser D, Schenk RK, Steinmann S, Fiorellini JP, Fox CH, Stich H: Influence of surface characteristics on bone integration of titanium implants—a histomorphometric study in miniature pigs. J Biomed Mater Res 1991, 25:889–902.

[33] Wong M, Eulenberger J, Schenk R, Hunziker E. Effect of surface topology on the osseointegration of implant materials in trabecular bone. J Biomed Mater Res 1995, 29:1567–1575.

[34] Wennerberg A, Ektessabi A, Albrektsson T, Johansson L, Andersson B: A 1-year follow-up of implants of differing surface roughness placed in rabbit bone. Int J Oral Max Implants 1997, 12:486–494.

[35] Boyan BD, Batzer R, Kieswetter K, Liu Y, Cochran DL, Szmuckler-Moncler SS, Dean DD, Schwartz Z: Titanium surface roughness alters responsiveness of MG63 osteoblast-like cells to 1 alpha,25-(OH)(2)D3. J Biomed Mater Res 1998, 39:77–85.

[36] Buchanan RA, Lee IS, Williams JM: Surface modification of biomaterials through noble metal ion implantation. J Biomed Mater Res 1990, 24:309–318.

[37] Sioshansi P: Surface modification of industrial components by ion implantation. Mater Sci Eng 1987, 90:373-383.

[38] Bauerle D: Laser processing and chemistry. Berlin, Heidelberg, New York, Tokyo: Springer; 2000

[39] Gaggl A, Schultes G, Müller WD, Kärcher H: Scanning electron microscopical analysis of lasertreated titanium implant surfaces - a comparative study. Biomaterials 2000; 21:1067–1073.

[40] György E, Mihailescu IN, Serra P, Pérez del Pino A, Morenza JL: Crown-like structure development on titanium exposed to multipulse NdYAG laser irradiation. Appl Phys A 2002; 74:755–759.

[41] Bereznai M, Pelsőczi I, Tóth Z, Turzó K, Radnai M, Bor Z, Fazekas A: Surface modifications induced by ns and sub-ps excimer laser pulses on titanium implant material. Biomaterials 2003, 24:4197-4203.

[42] Sun L, Berndt CC, Gross KA, Kucuk A: Material fundamentals and clinical performance of plasmasprayed hydroxyapatite coatings: a review. J Biomed Mater Res 2001, 58:570-592.

[43] Rohanizadeh R, LeGeros RZ, Harsono M, Bendavid A. Adherent apatite coating on titanium substrate using chemical deposition. J Biomed Mater Res A 2005, 72:428-438.

[44] Block M, Gardiner D, Kent J, Misiek D, Finger I, Guerra L: Hydroxyapatite-coated cylinder implants in the posterior mandible: 10 years observations. Int J Oral Maxillofac Implants 1996, 11:626-633.

[45] Buser D, Schenk RK, Steinemann S, Fiorellini JP, Fox CH, Stich H: Influence of surface characteristics on bone integration of titanium implants. A histometric study in miniature pigs. J Biomed Mater Res 1991, 25:889-902.

[46] Matsui Y, Ohno K, Michi K, Yamagata K: Experimental study of high velocity flame-sprayed hydroxyapatite coated and noncoated titanium implants. Int J Oral Maxillofac Implants 1994, 9:397-404.

[47] Wheeler SL: Eight-year clinical retrospective study of titanium plasma-sprayed and hydroxyapatitecoated cylinder implants. Int J Oral Maxillofac Implants 1996, 11:340-350.

[48] de Jonge LT, Leeuwenburgh SCG, Wolke JGC, Jansen JA: Organic-inorganic surface modifications for titanium implant surfaces. Pharmaceutical Research 2008, DOI: 10.1007/s11095-008-9617-0.

[49] Sykaras N, Opperman LA: Bone morphogenetic proteins (BMPs): how do they function and what can they offer the clinician? Journal of Oral Science 2003, 2:57-73.

[50] Liu Y, de Groot K, Hunziker EB: BMP-2 liberated from biomimetic implant coatings induces and sustains direct ossification in an ectopic rat model. Bone 2005, 36:745-757.

[51] Nickel J, Dreyer MK, Kirsch T, Sebald W: The crystal structure of the BMP-2: BMPR-IA complex and the generation of BMP-2 antagonists. J Bone Joint Surg AM 2001, 83A:S7-S14.

[52] Urist MR: Bone: formation by autoinduction. Science 1965, 150:893-9.

[53] Sakou T: Bone morphogenetic proteins: from basic studies to clinical approaches. Bone 1998, 22:591- 603.

[54] Ferris DM, Moodie GD, Dimond PM, Gioranni CW, Ehrlich GM, Valentini RF: RGD-coated titanium implants stimulate increased bone formation in vivo. Biomaterials 1999, 20:2323-2331.

[55] Schliephake H, Scharnweber D, Dard M, Sewing A, Aref A, Roessler S: Functionalization of dental implant surfaces using adhesion molecules. J Biomed Mater Res B Appl. Biomater 2005, 73:88-96.

[56] Pelsőczi I, Turzó K, Gergely C, Fazekas A, Dékány I, Cuisinier F: Structural characterization of selfassembled polypeptide films on titanium and glass surfaces by atomic force microscopy. Biomacromolecules 2005, 6:3345-3350.

[57] van den Beucken JJ, Walboomers XF, Leeuwenburgh SC, Vos MR, Sommerdijk NA, Nolte RJ, Jansen JA: Multilayered DNA coatings: in vitro bioactivity studies and effects on osteoblast-like cell behavior. Acta Biomater 2007, 3:587-596.

[58] Golub EE, Boesze-Battaglia K: The role of alkaline phosphatase in mineralization. Curr. Opin. Orthop 2007, 18:444-448.

[59] Morra M, Cassinelli C, Cascardo G, Cahalan P, Cahalan L, Fini M, Giardino R: Surface engineering of titanium by collagen immobilization. Surface characterization and in vitro and in vivo studies. Biomaterials 2003, 24:4639-4654.

[60] Liu Y, Huse RO, de Groot K, Buser D, Hunziker EB. Delivery mode and efficacy of BMP-2 in association with implants. J Dent Res 2007, 86:84-89.

[61] Sikirić MD, Gergely C, Elkaim R, Wachtel E, Cuisinier FJ, Füredi-Milhofer H: Biomimetic organicinorganic nanocomposite coatings for titanium implants. J Biomed Mater Res A, 2008 May 8. DOI: 10.1002/jbm.a.32021.

[62] Johnston MC, Bronsky PT: Animal models for human craniofacial malformations J.Craniofac. Genet. Dev. Biol., 1991, 11:277–291

[63] Hau J, Van Hoosier GL, Svendsen P, Van Hoosier GL Jr.: Handbook of Laboratory Animal Science, 2002.

[64] Baron M, Haas R, Dortbudak O, Watzek G. Experimentally induced peri-implantitis: a review of different treatment methods described in the literature. Int J Oral Maxillofac Implants. 2000, 15:533-44.

[65] Caiazza S, Colangelo P, Bedini R, Formisano G, De Angelis G, Barrucci S. Evaluation of guided bone regeneration in rabbit femur using collagen membranes. Implant Dent. 2000, 9(3):219-25.

[66] Fialkov JA, Holy CE, Shoichet MS, Davies JE.: In Vivo Bone Engineering in a Rabbit Femur. The Journal of Craniofacial Surgery 2003, 14: 324–332.

[67] Bidic SMS, Calvert JW, Marra K, Kumta P, Campbell P, Mitchell R, Wigginton W, Hollinger JO, Weiss L, Mooney MP: Rabbit Calvarial Wound Healing by Means of Seeded Caprotite® Scaffolds, Journal of Dental Research, 2003, 82:131-135.

[68] Schantz JT, Hutmacher DW, Lam CXF, Brinkmann M, Wong KM, Lim TC, Chou N, Guldberg RE, Teoh SH: Repair of Calvarial Defects with Customised Tissue-Engineered Bone Grafts and Evaluation of Cellular Efficiency and Efficacy in Vivo, Tissue Engineering. 2003, 9:127-139.

[69] Gosain AK, Song L, Yu P, Mehrara BJ, Maeda CY, Gold LI, Longaker MT: Quantitative Assessment of Cranial Defect Healing and Correlation with the Expression of TGF-β, Journal of Craniofacial Surgery. 2001, 12:401-404.

[70] Springer I, Açil Y, Kuchenbecker S, Bolte H, Warnke P, Abboud M, Wiltfang J, Terheyden H: Bone graft versus BMP-7 in a critical size defect—Cranioplasty in a growing infant model. Bone. 37:563-569.

[71] Artzi Z, Givol N, Rohrer MD, Nemcovsky CE, Prasad HS, Tal H. Qualitative and quantitative expression of bovine bone mineral in experimental bone defects. Part 2: Morphometric analysis. J Periodontol. 2003, 74:1153-60.

[72] Conner KA, Sabatini R, Mealey BL, Takacs VJ, Mills MP, Cochran DL. Guided bone regeneration around titanium plasma-sprayed, acid-etched, and hydroxyapatite-coated implants in the canine model. J Periodontol. 2003, 74:658-68.

YOUR KNOWLEDGE HAS VALUE

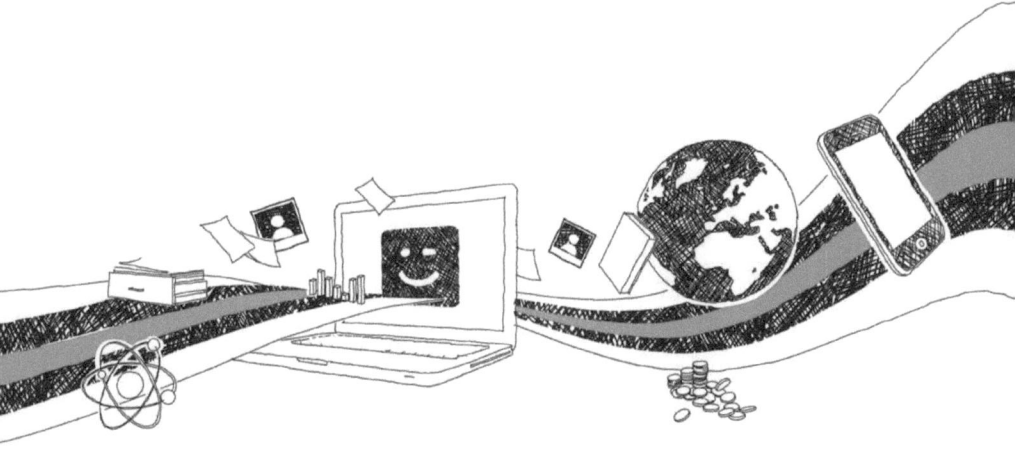

- We will publish your bachelor's and
  master's thesis, essays and papers

- Your own eBook and book -
  sold worldwide in all relevant shops

- Earn money with each sale

Upload your text at www.GRIN.com
and publish for free

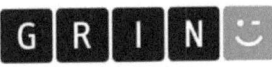